# VAGINAL YEAST INFECTION

TREATMENTS STRATEGIES FOR VAGINAL
YEAST INFECTION

**DR. KATE .P**

# Contents

# CHAPTER ONE

## INTRODUCTION

One kind of vaginal inflammation known as vaginitis, which is characterized by vaginal irritation, severe itching, and vaginal discharge, is a vaginal yeast infection. Your vagina and the tissues surrounding its opening are impacted by a vaginal yeast infection (vulva).

Vaginal candidiasis, another name for vaginal yeast infection, is extremely frequent. Yeast infections affect up to three out of every four women at some point in their lives. Many women get at least one yeast infection.

Even while the fungus that causes vaginal yeast infections can be transferred from oral to genital contact, the illness is not regarded as sexually transmitted. Unless you have four or more recurrent yeast infections in a single year, simple therapy is usually sufficient. If so, you could require a longer therapy session as well as a maintenance schedule.

## Symptoms

Symptoms of a yeast infection can be mild to moderate and include:

Itching and discomfort near the vulva's entrance as well as inside the vagina a scorching feeling, particularly when urinating or having sex

**Vulva's redness and swelling**

Pain and soreness in the vagina

thick, white, odorless vaginal discharge that resembles cottage cheese

complex yeast infection

A complex yeast infection may be present in you if:

You exhibit severe symptoms, including widespread redness, swelling, and itching that causes tears, fissures, or sores to appear.

You have four or more recurring yeast infections in a single year.

Other than Candida albicans, another form of candida is the source of your problem.

It's you who's expecting

You have diabetes that is out of control.

Because of the usage of some medications or a medical condition like HIV infection, your immunity has decreased.

## When to visit a physician

Schedule a visit with your physician if:

You've never had signs of a yeast infection before.

It's unclear if you have a yeast infection.

After self-treating with over-the-counter antifungal vaginal creams or suppositories, your symptoms don't go away

You experience additional symptoms.

### Reasons

The fungal infection candida is the source of a vaginal yeast infection. Along with bacteria, candida is a type of microbe that is typically found in the vagina. There is a healthy balance of bacteria and yeast in your vagina by nature. Acid produced by Lactobacillus bacteria prevents yeast from growing too much in the vagina. However, an excess of yeast might arise from a disturbance of the delicate equilibrium. Yeast infection symptoms such as burning and itching in the vagina can be caused by an overabundance of yeast in the vagina.

**Yeast overgrowth may arise from:**

Use of antibiotics causes the lactobacillus bacteria in your vagina to diminish and alters the pH of your vagina, allowing yeast to overgrow

Being pregnant

Unmanaged diabetes

compromised immune system

Anything, such douching or irritation from insufficient vaginal lubrication, that modifies the kind and quantity of bacteria typically found in the vagina

Candida albicans is a form of candida fungus that typically causes yeast infections. However, symptoms may occasionally be caused by a different kind of candida fungus. Typical therapies for yeast infections are effective in treating Candida albicans. However, some forms of candida may not react well to standard treatments and may need more intensive care.

It is possible to contract a yeast infection through intercourse, particularly oral-genital contact. Since the candida fungus is normally found in the vagina and yeast infections occur in women who are not sexually active, they are not classified as STDs.

# RISK ELEMENTS

The following variables raise your chance of getting a yeast infection:

usage of antibiotics. Women who use antibiotics are more likely to get yeast infections. Antibiotics that are effective against a broad spectrum of germs, or broad-spectrum antibiotics, destroy good bacteria in your vagina and can cause an overgrowth of yeast.

elevated amounts of estrogen. Women with elevated estrogen levels, such as those who are pregnant, on high-dose estrogen birth control pills, or undergoing estrogen hormone therapy, seem to be more susceptible to yeast infections.

unmanaged diabetes. Compared to women whose diabetes is under control, women with diabetes who have poorly regulated blood sugar levels are more likely to experience yeast infections.

compromised immune system. Yeast infections are more common in women who have compromised immune systems, such as those caused by corticosteroid medication or HIV infection.

Intercourse. Sexual intercourse is one method through which the candida organism can enter your vagina, even though yeast infections are not classified as STDs.

# Getting Ready for Your Consultation

Your doctor might be able to prescribe a prescription over the phone and avoid a visit if you have previously received treatment for a yeast infection. If not, your gynecologist or family doctor will probably treat your issue.

## What you're capable of

Do not use tampons or douche before your appointment so that your doctor can see and assess your vaginal discharge.

Here are some details to help you get ready for your visit and understand what to anticipate from your physician.

Jot down any symptoms you've experienced, along with their duration.

Important medical information should be noted, such as any additional conditions you are being treated for and the names of any prescription drugs, vitamins, or supplements you are taking.

In order to allow your doctor to analyze any vaginal discharge you may have, avoid using tampons or douching before your consultation.

In the event that you are pressed for time, prioritize your list of questions for your doctor.

Some fundamental inquiries for your doctor regarding a yeast infection are as follows:

How can yeast infections be avoided?

Which symptoms and indicators should I be aware of?

Should I take medication?

Does testing or treatment for my partner also need to be done?

Are there any specific directions on how to take the medication?

Exist any over-the-counter medications that can help with my condition?

What should I do if, following treatment, my symptoms come back?

Do not be afraid to ask additional questions as they come to mind throughout your visit.

You should expect to be asked a lot of questions by your doctor, including:

Which symptoms are related to vagina?

Does your vagina seem particularly stinky?

What is the duration of your symptoms?

Have you ever had a vaginal infection treated?

Have you attempted any over-the-counter remedies for your ailment?

Have you taken any antibiotics recently?

Do you engage in sexual activity?

Do you have a baby?

Do you take bubble baths or use scented soap?

Do you use feminine hygiene spray or are you a douche?

Which prescription drugs or dietary supplements do you take on a daily basis?



If your doctor suspects a yeast infection, they might:

Inquire about your past medical records. Information regarding previous vaginal infections or STDs may be gathered in this way.

Do a pelvic examination. the external genitalia are visually inspected by the doctor to look for infection symptoms. Then, in order to check the

16

vagina and cervix, your doctor will insert a device called a speculum into your vagina to hold the walls open. If a vaginal culture test is required, your doctor may take a sample of any vaginal discharge for examination under a microscope.

For testing, send in a sample of vaginal secretions. Your doctor most likely won't order any blood work for simple yeast infections. However, if your doctor is aware of the particular type of yeast that is causing your illness, they might be able to recommend a more successful course of therapy if you have recurrent yeast infections.

# CHAPTER TWO

## MEDICATIONS AND SUBTLES

The course of treatment for a yeast infection varies depending on how simple or complicated the infection is.

Simple yeast infection

Your doctor may suggest the following for occasional occurrences of a yeast infection with mild to moderate symptoms:

brief vaginal treatment. Most of the time, a yeast infection can be successfully treated with a single application or a one-to three-day regimen of an antifungal cream, ointment, pill, or suppository. The preferred drug is from the azole class, which also includes clotrimazole (Gyne-Lotrimin), miconazole (Monistat 3), terconazole (Terazol 3), and butoconazole (Gynazole-1). These drugs can be purchased over-the-counter or with a prescription. These agents' oil-based composition in cream and suppository form may make latex condoms and diaphragms less effective. Slight stinging or discomfort upon application are possible side effects.

oral medicine taken once. Your doctor may recommend taking the antifungal drug fluconazole (Diflucan) orally once in a single dose.

If your symptoms have not improved after your treatment has ended or if they reappear within two months of starting treatment, schedule a follow-up visit with your doctor.

complex yeast infection

An intricate yeast infection may be treated with one of the following:

long-term vaginal treatment. An azole medicine administered as a vaginal cream, ointment, pill, or suppository is one of the vaginal treatments for complex yeast infections. Typically, the course of treatment lasts seven to fourteen days.

oral medicine administered in multiple doses. Your doctor may recommend taking fluconazole orally in two or three doses as an alternative to vaginal therapy. Pregnant women are not advised to have this therapy, nevertheless.

Plan of maintenance. Your doctor may suggest a drug regimen to control yeast overgrowth and stop further infections if you have recurrent yeast infections. After the initial course of treatment resolves the yeast infection, maintenance therapy may involve taking fluconazole tablets orally once a week for a period of six months. Instead of giving patients an oral prescription, some doctors prescribe clotrimazole as a vaginal pill, or suppository, to be administered once a week.

Most of the time, treating your sex partner's yeast infection does not also need to be done. Your doctor may advise treating your partner if they exhibit symptoms of a genital yeast infection, such as jock itch in a male partner, or they may advise using condoms during sexual activity if you have recurring yeast infections.

## WAY OF LIFE AND DOMESTIC MEDICINE

To lower the chance of getting a vaginal yeast infection:

Refrain from douching.

Wear loose-fitting skirts or pants and cotton underwear.

Steer clear of pantyhose or tight-fitting underwear.

As soon as you can, change out of damp clothing, such as swimsuits or exercise gear.

Avoid taking very hot baths or hot tubs.

## OTHER FORM OF MEDICINE

While some research has been done on alternative treatments for yeast infections, more well planned and regulated trials are required to fully understand these treatments before professionals can offer any advice.

As examples, consider:

acid boric. If you have persistent (chronic) symptoms that don't go away or recurring yeast infections, boric acid, a prescription vaginal insert (suppository), may be a good substitute for traditional therapy. When it comes to less prevalent strains of candida and candida that has developed resistance to azole medicines, boric acid may be useful. However, boric acid is dangerous if swallowed accidently, especially by young children, and it can cause skin irritation.

yogurt. Anecdotally, some women claim success when using yogurt that contains lactobacillus, either topically or orally. That being said, this strategy is still unproven. Research demonstrating the efficacy of yogurt in lowering vaginal yeast cultures and relieving symptoms was conducted on a limited number of women without the presence of control groups. Those findings have not been supported by additional research.

Discuss the advantages and disadvantages of any alternative therapy with your doctor before attempting any.

**THE END**